THE ANTI-CANCER LIFESTYLE

METHODS TO REDUCE RISK AND IMPROVE HEALTH

BY

DR. SHARON COLSON

INTRODUCTION

"The Anti-Cancer Lifestyle" is a book that aims to guide readers toward a cancer-free future by emphasizing health and wellbeing.

It places a strong emphasis on wellbeing from all angles, including diet, mindfulness, stress reduction, exercise, rest, and movement.

The book promotes holistic treatment, which includes complementary therapies and herbal cures, and analyzes the effects of the environment on health. Not only are facts and data important, but also empowerment, educated choice-making, and the development of a lifestyle that lowers the risk of cancer and improves general quality of life.

Join the quest towards a world free of cancer.

CHAPTER ONE

UNDERSTANDING CANCER RISK

Risk is the chance that an event will occur. "Cancer threat" is most frequently used to describe the chance that a person will develop cancer.

In cancer care, this expression is also used to describe the chance that the cancer will come back after treatment. When cancer returns, it's called a rush.

Exploring the cancer threat helps ameliorate the health of numerous people. For illustration, when scientists discovered that smoking increases the threat of lung cancer,anti-smoking juggernauts began and have helped save numerous lives.

It's also important for people to understand the particular threat of developing cancer. Knowing your individual threat factors can help you form opinions about your health and habits that can reduce your threat of developing cancer and/or increase your chance of catching cancer at an earlier stage.

Cancer that's set up at an earlier stage may be easier to treat or have a better prognostic.

The Difference Between An Absolute Threat and A Relative Threat

Croakers and experimenters use two different threat factor computations to understand the cancer threat:

The absolute threat and the relative threat.

Understanding absolute threat and relative threat can help you get a clear picture of your particular threat, which can help you form health care and life opinions.

The absolute threat tells you the average person's chance of developing cancer during a specific period of time. For illustration, the continued threat of an average person developing colorectal cancer is around 4.1. In other words, about 1 in 24 people will develop colorectal cancer in their lifetime.

An absolute threat cannot tell you the threat to a specific person or a specific group of people.

Relative threat compares one group's threat of developing cancer with another group's. For illustration, exploration shows that people with diabetes have a 38-year-old advanced threat of developing colorectal cancer.

It's important to remember that this doesn't mean that a person with diabetes has a 38 percent chance of developing colorectal cancer in the future. It means that there's a 38 percent increase over the absolute threat (4.1).

The increase in the threat for a person with diabetes of developing colorectal cancer is 1.6, which means their continued threat is 5.7.

To calculate the increase in absolute threat in this specific illustration, you first need to find out what 38 of 4.1 is. You can do this by converting the probabilities to numbers: 0.38 x 0.041 =.016. also add together the original absolute threat (4.1) and the increase in threat (1.6) to get the new continuance threat of 5.7.

Both absolute and relative threats are important when you're considering your own threat of developing cancer. You can use these threat measures to know if or when you need certain types of cancer webbing or to make healthy life choices.

However, make sure you find the data about the increase in absolute threat if you want to compare any exploration you hear about in the news to your own situation.

Most exploration studies and news stories report a relative threat. This can make it feel like your threat of developing cancer is more advanced than it actually is.

And always talk with your croaker about what you're hearing about cancer threats and about your particular cancer threat. Ask about any new terms that you do not understand.

This helps you have clear information about your cancer threat and your croaker.

Your health care plan can also guide you toward similar healthy habits, such as how to quit smoking, get regular exercise, and eat healthy foods.

What are common cancer threat factors?

A cancer threat factor is anything that increases a person's threat of developing cancer.

Most threat factors don't directly cause cancer. Having a threat factor doesn't mean that you will surely develop cancer.

Some people with several risk factors never develop cancer. And others with no known threat factors do. It's important to know your threat factors and talk about them with your health care team.

Knowing this information can help you make medical and life choices to improve your health. It can also help your health care plan decide if you need inheritable testing and comforting.

General threat factors for cancer includes;

- Aging
- A particular or family history of cancer, using tobacco, carrying too much weight, known as being fat

- Alcohol use
- Some types of viral infections, such as mortal papillomavirus(HPV) and hepatitis contagion.
- Exposure to specific chemicals.
- Exposure to radiation, including ultraviolet radiation from the sun.

Some threat factors can be avoided or used in temperance. Other threat factors cannot be avoided, such as getting older. It's important to remember that it isn't just the type of threat factor, it is the quantum of exposure, how frequently, and when the exposure happens.

For illustration, weight gain after menopause is linked to an advanced bone cancer threat.

The listed particulars above aren't the only threat factors for cancer. There are more specific risk factors for specific types of cancer.

The likelihood of discovering cancer or precancerous spots while they are smaller and often simpler to treat improves with screening.

If you have a high chance of getting cancer, surgery or medication may be able to reduce that risk. For instance, some individuals are more likely to have breast cancer if their mother, father, or another close relative did.

Some individuals have long family histories of breast cancer or genetic abnormalities connected to the disease. They may decide to undergo surgery to remove their breasts in order to avoid cancer, since they have a very high chance of developing breast cancer.

The chance of developing breast cancer seems to be reduced by at least 95% after this operation. They may also decide to take medications to reduce their chance of developing breast cancer.

People who are worried about a cancer history in their family can consider genetic testing. You may discuss having specific genetic testing with your doctor or a genetic counselor.

Based on your family history and other risk factors, they may inform you of your likelihood of developing cancer.

CHAPTER TWO

FOODS THAT FIGHT CANCER AND PREVENT IT

When you have cancer, your cells' DNA and genes get destroyed, causing the cells to begin to mutate and expand out of control.

Cancer cells, in contrast to healthy cells, develop immortality and begin quickly spreading throughout the body, consuming all of your nutrition and depleting your sugar supply.

As the cells change, they create tumors that lead to cancer in several organs, including your bowels. For instance, the liver, pancreas, or lungs.

Your nerves are also destroyed by cancerous cells, your organs and blood vessels, and finally result in death.

What, however, really harms your DNA and cells in the first place?

The frequent addition of refined sugar to our diets is one of the key culprits as the mitochondria within your cells get damaged by free radicals as a result.

High-fructose corn syrup is another substance that increases the risk of cancer utilized in the production of fast food, sauces, juice drinks, and confectionery.

Even the aspartame-based artificial sweeteners used in diet drinks your cells' insulin receptors, which may potentially result in cancer.

Vegetable oils that have been refined also cause cancer.

Processed grains and wheat that deplete your antioxidant reserves and increase your risk of DNA damage

Additionally, the chemical weed killers and pesticides used to cultivate our vegetables are damaging to your cells. Along with drinking alcohol, vaping, smoking, and other breathing contaminants,

Thankfully, there are natural foods with curative qualities which aid in preventing cancer in your cells.

Raw Garlic

Regular use of raw, crushed garlic may assist in preventing the development of malignant cells in your body.

It includes organic compounds including ajoene, allicin, and sulfur that increase

Antioxidant activity in your body guards against cellular, mitochondrial, and DNA deterioration.

Garlic's allicin has also been shown to aggravate pre-existing the self-destruction and death of cancer cells (apoptosis).

Crushing your garlic is essential to releasing allicin, and be careful not to fry it since heat can ruin this delicate composition.

Broccoli sprouts

Sprouts of broccoli are 2-3 days old microgreens that have been grown from broccoli seeds for a day. Sulforaphane, an anti-cancer substance, is abundant in them.

This keeps your good cells intact while causing the suicide of malignant cells.

Sulforaphane levels in broccoli sprouts are 100 times higher than in mature broccoli.

More enzymes are produced by your liver to help your body eliminate poisons and pollutants(That may have, over time, led to cancer.)

These are fairly simple to begin cultivating at home.

You can grow sprouts for cheap on your windowsill.

Cauliflower, radish, and other wheatgrass seeds or arugula seeds may also be consumed since they contain anti-cancer chemicals.

They may be added on top of the cooked veggies, since the enzymes therein aid in increasing the amount of nutrients your stomach can absorb from cooked meals.

Or you may just mix them into a nutritious salad.

Blueberries

Begin consuming a small handful of blueberries daily to boost your immune system and general wellness.

Anthocyanins are plant pigments found in blueberries and other berries. They are black, purple, or reddish coloring.

Strong antioxidants called anthocyanins protect your cells against oxidative stress that is brought on by sugar, processed meals, vegetable oils, etc.

If you want to keep your body from getting hurt or recovering from any illnesses, you need to concentrate on consuming meals high in antioxidants every day.

Bilberries, blackberries, strawberries, and raspberries are further cancer-fighting berries.

Some of the acai and gooseberries may be consumed as a powdered supplement.

Savoy cabbage

A form of fermented cabbage popular in Germany is called sauerkraut.

It is one of the world's greatest sources of vitamin C.

700 mg of vitamin C, or more than 8 times the daily amount, may be found in 1 cup.

Areas of your body that are swollen and inflamed are common places for cancer to spread.

However, vitamin C aids in reducing this irritation, and eliminate free radicals from your blood to lower your chance of developing cancer.

You should consume foods high in the real vitamin C complex.

Supplemental "ascorbic acid" does not have the same impact as whole meals do.

Due to fermentation, it contains a lot of probiotics and prebiotics, which are beneficial microorganisms.

It help nourish the cells in your colon and stop the development of polyps, tumors, and bowel cancer.

Kimchi, miso, kefir, and plain Greek yogurt (full fat) are other fantastic fermented foods.

Fruits and vegetables

Many of us have mistreated our bodies for a long time consuming a lot of sweets, junk food, and possibly alcohol.

Toxins may accumulate as a result in the liver, bones, and other organs and tissues that might increase your chance of developing cancer in the future.

Fortunately, you can assist your body in beginning to eliminate these by consuming a lot of organic cruciferous veggies, which are free of carcinogens.

Brussels sprouts, broccoli, cauliflower, kale, and beet tops, for example; Watercress, bok choy, arugula, collard greens, etc.

These brassica vegetables are loaded with anti-cancer nutrients. In addition to vitamin C, potassium, magnesium, B vitamins, and many more nutrients

These nutrients support the breakdown of poisons by liver enzymes, which harmless water-soluble particles that your urine may discharge.

Phase 1 and Phase 2 detoxification are used to describe this.

You may softly steam your veggies, but be careful not to overcook them.

In a salad with other vegetables like tomatoes, spring onions, herbs, etc., it is recommended to consume them raw.

Pepper and turmeric

One of the most well-known natural remedies is turmeric medications for reducing inflammation and promoting the body's natural healing processes.

Start incorporating turmeric powder into stir-fries, curries, and other dishes.

It may be used to create herbal tea, soups, or stews.

Curcumin is the name of turmeric's active component.

Recent research indicates that it inhibits the development of new blood vessels in malignant tumors.

This aids in starving cancer cells and halts the progression of malignancy.

Every time you consume turmeric, you should also add black pepper because it includes piperine, which may increase your ability to absorb curcumin by 2000%.

Mushrooms

Turkey tail, shiitake, and maitake are some of the top mushrooms for fighting cancer.

Maitake, reishi, lion's mane, cordyceps, and chaga

These in fact include more than 40 distinct phytonutrients that aid in the prevention and treatment of cancer like baicalein, hispolon, quercetin, and many more.

Matcha Green Tea

If you're serious about enhancing your family's health, begin ingesting 2 cups of matcha green tea every day.

Unlike normal green tea, Matcha offers more concentrated nutrients with therapeutic qualities and more chlorophyll than other teas.

Its main ingredient, EGCG, has shown the ability to inhibit the growth of cancer cells, preventing a tumor's ability to spread to the body's tissues and organs.

Wild Fish Caught

Typically, injured and inflamed bodily regions are where cancer originates and spreads.

Consequently, it's crucial to keep inflammation under control.

This will lessen the possibility of getting cancer and aid in the battle against it.

Wild fish like sardines, salmon, and mackerel are some of the most effective anti-inflammatory nutrients.

DHA and EPA, two active omega-3 fatty acids found in this fish, aid in reducing swelling and inflammation against cancer's damaging effects.

Eat these foods as directed by your doctor if you're on a cancer treatment regimen, often to aid your body in adjusting to the chemotherapy treatments and therapies.

You may consume 500 mg of Antarctic Krill Oil each day as a supplement. It contains a lot of stable omega-3s.

It also includes astaxanthin, a potent antioxidant and carotenoid that fights cancer.

Dark chocolate without added sugar

The cacao beans used to produce chocolate are loaded with phytonutrients and antioxidants such as chlorogenic acid, which has also been shown to prevent cancer.

In fact, it has more flavonols than blueberries and acai; therefore, adding this to your routine is an excellent way to increase the body's supply of antioxidants.

Make sure you choose a dark beverage that is mostly organic.

Stevia, rather than sugar, is used to sweeten chocolate (at least 70% cocoa solids).

Consuming a few cubes daily might help manage blood pressure reduce cortisol, the stress hormone that causes weight gain, and decrease cholesterol.

CHAPTER THREE

CANCER-CAUSING FOODS

Do you know that the food you eat could be adding to your risk of cancer? It's not just genetics or life choices but also the foods we consume that can contribute to this deadly complaint.

Certain foods have been linked to an increased threat of cancer, while genetics and life choices can also play a part in the development of cancer. The foods we eat can contribute to this complaint as well.

Some foods contain dangerous chemicals or composites that have been linked to cancer, While others can promote inflammation or contribute to the development of cancer

In other ways, it's important to be apprehensive of these cancer-causing foods and to make healthy nutritional choices in order to reduce your threat of developing this ruinous complaint.

- **Reused fabric Flesh-like bacon bangers**

Hot tykes and deli flesh have been linked to an increased threat of several types of cancer, including colorectal, stomach, and pancreatic cancer.

These tykes contain dangerous chemicals like nitrates and nitrites, which can form cancer-causing composites when consumed

In addition, they're frequently high in sodium and impregnated fat, which can also contribute to cancer development.

It's stylish to limit your input of reused flesh or avoid them all together and choose healthier protein sources like spare flesh fish and factory-ground options.

- **Fried Foods**

Fried foods like French Feast, fried funk, and donuts have been linked to an increased threat of several types of cancer.

When foods are fried at high temperatures, dangerous composites like acrylamide can form.

Acrylamide has been linked to an increased threat of several types of cancer, including ovarian and pancreatic cancer.

In addition, fried foods are frequently high in unhealthy fats and calories, which can contribute to rotundity and other health issues that increase the threat of cancer.

It's stylish to limit your consumption of fried foods and choose healthier cuisine styles like incinerating grilling or sautéing.

- **Sugar**

A diet high in sugar has been linked to several types of cancer, including bone ovarian and colorectal cancer.

Sugar can also promote inflammation in the body, which can contribute to the development of cancer.

When we consume too much sugar, our bodies release more insulin, which can stimulate the growth of cancer cells.

It's important to be aware of your sugar intake and try to limit your consumption of sticky foods and drinks like soda pop delicacies and ignited goods.

Instead, choose whole foods like fruits, vegetables, and whole grains, which contain natural sugars and provide important nutrients and fiber that can help reduce the threat of cancer.

- **Acohol**

Drinking alcohol has been linked to an increased threat of several types of cancer, including bone, liver, and colorectal cancer.

When we consume alcohol, our bodies break it down into a dangerous chemical called acetaldehyde, which can damage DNA and increase the threat of cancer development.

In addition, alcohol can also contribute to the production of free radicals, which can damage cells and increase the threat of cancer.

It's stylish to limit your alcohol consumption or avoid it all together.

The American Cancer Society recommends that women have no more than one drink per day, and men have no more than two drinks per day.

- **Artificial Sweeteners**

Artificial sweeteners like aspartame, saccharin, and sucrose have been the subject of controversy regarding their implicit links to cancer.

While studies haven't set up conclusive substantiation that artificial sweeteners cause cancer in humans, some studies in rodents have suggested a possible link.

In addition, artificial sweeteners can contribute to other health issues like diabetes and rotundity, which are also risk factors for cancer.

If you're looking for a sweetener, consider using natural sweeteners like honey, maple syrup, saccharinity, or stevia, which are less reused and may be a safer option.

Still, it's important to consume sweeteners in moderation and be aware of your overall sugar input.

- **Soda pop**

Soda pop and other sticky drinks like sports drinks and energy drinks have been linked to an increased threat of several types of cancer, including bone, colorectal, and pancreatic cancer.

These drinks are high in sugar and calories, which can contribute to rotundity and other health issues that increase the threat of cancer.

In addition, soda pop frequently contains dangerous chemicals like caramel color and methylamidazole for Mei, which have been linked to cancer development.

It's stylish to limit your consumption of sticky drinks and choose healthier options like water, thin tea, or low-fat milk.

- **Hydrogenated Canvases**

Hydrogenated canvases, also known as trans fats, have been linked to an increased threat of several types of cancer, including gut and colorectal cancer.

These canvases are generally set up with reused foods, like ignited goods, fried foods and snacks.

Hydrogenation is a process that turns liquid canvases into solids, making them more stable and adding to their shelf life.

During the hydrogenation process, dangerous trans fats are formed. These trans fats can increase

LDL-bad cholesterol levels and promote inflammation, both of which can contribute to cancer development.

It's stylish to avoid foods that contain hydrogenated canvases and choose healthier options like foods made with healthy fats, such as olive oil, avocado, and nuts.

- **White-flour foods**

White-flour foods made with white flour, similar to white chuck and pasta have been linked to an increased threat of several types of cancer, including colorectal cancer.

This is because white flour is heavily reused and stripped of its nutrients and fiber, which can contribute to inflammation and other health issues that increase the threat of cancer.

In addition, white flour is frequently added to reused foods like crackers, eyefuls, and galettes, which can further increase the threat of cancer.

It's stylish to choose whole-grain alternatives like whole-wheat chuck.and pasta, which are rich in nutrients and fiber that can help reduce inflammation and promote good health.

- **Red meat**

Red meat, including beef, pork, and chicken, has been linked to an increased threat of several types of cancer, including colorectal, pancreatic, and prostate cancer.

This is because red meat contains a high amount of impregnated fat, which can contribute to inflammation and increase the threat of cancer development.

In addition, red meat also contains brim iron, which can damage the filling of the colon and increase the threat of colorectal cancer.

It's stylish to limit your consumption of red meat and choose slender protein sources like fish funk or factory-ground proteins like sap and legumes.

If you do consume red meat, it's important to choose spare cuts and cook them using healthy styles like grilling or broiling, and avoid reusing. Flesh like bacon and links have been linked to an increased threat of cancer.

- **Canned foods**

Canning foods, particularly those that are acidic, have been linked to an increased threat of cancer. This is because the filling of most mimetic foods contains bisphenolate BPA, a chemical that can strain into the food and disrupt hormone function, potentially leading to the development of cancer

Canned foods that are particularly high in acidity, such as tomatoes and citrus fruits, can increase the threat of BPA filtering into the food.

In addition, canned foods may also contain preservatives and complements that can contribute to cancer development.

It's stylish to choose fresh or frozen fruits and vegetables over mimetic options. If you do choose canned foods, look for BPA-free options or those that are canned in glass jars.

- **Dairy products**

Dairy products such as milk and yogurt have been linked to an increased threat of several types of cancer, including bone ovarian and prostate cancer. This is because dairy products contain hormones similar to estrogen, which can promote cancer growth.

In addition, some dairy products, particularly those that are high in impregnated fat, can contribute to inflammation and increase the threat of cancer development.

Still, it's important to note that some studies have suggested that consuming low-fat dairy products may actually reduce the threat of certain types of cancer.

It's stylish to choose low-fat dairy products. Limit your consumption of high-fat dairy products and opt for factory-ground milk.

- **Grilled vegetables**

Grilled vegetables are generally considered a healthy food option as they're high in nutrients and fiber and low in calories. Still, there are some concerns about the implicit cancer-causing effects of grilling food, including vegetables.

When food is grilled at high temperatures, it can produce chemicals called heterocyclic amines (HCAS) and polycyclic sweet hydrocarbons (PHS), which have been linked to an increased threat of cancer.

When grilling vegetables, it's important to cook them at a lower temperature and for a shorter time to avoid scorching or burning them.

Using gravies, particularly those containing ginger or citrus, can also help reduce the conformation of HCAS and PHS.

CHAPTER FOUR

CRUCIAL LIFESTYLE RECOMMENDATIONS TO PREVENT OR FIGHT CANCER

Given the wealth of knowledge you already possess about foods that prevent cancer, let's look at a few key lifestyle recommendations you may utilize to safeguard and repair your cells.

- Many patients have employed intermittent fasting for 48 hours or more to treat advanced cancer. IGF-1, glucose, insulin, and other substances increase during a fast. Growth factors are decreased, assisting the body in healing and eliminating cancer cells.
- Consuming soluble fiber-rich foods, such as chia seeds, helps nourish the good bacteria in the stomach. This increases the body's butyrate levels.

The body's overall inflammation is reduced as a result, and it inhibits oxidation, avoiding mitochondrial and cellular DNA damage.

- Cut down on consuming processed meats and dishes prepared in vegetable oil, and get rid of sugar in your system. By doing this, damage from free radicals to the cells will be reduced.

- Hydrate the body with at least 1 liter of mineral water daily, avoiding valve water, which contains hormone disruptors.

  You can also add potassium citrate to your water, which helps ameliorate cell function and removes redundant sugar in the blood.

- Focus on eating organic, antioxidant-rich foods formerly bandied to stimulate cellular mending.

  Add low-glycaemic berries, failures, krill oil painting, nutritive incentive, lawn-fed beef, organ flesh, and ocean kelp to your diet.

- Incipiently, get 20 twinkles of exercise at least twice per week. This increases oxygen levels by 10–20x in the blood. Cancer cells do not thrive in an oxygen-rich environment.

  Exercise outdoors when you can, as infrared light from the sun can boost melatonin, an important antioxidant.

  Also, be sure to quit smoking or vaping.

CHAPTER FIVE

FITNESS AND EXERCISE FOR CANCER DEFENSE

Exploration has shown that regular exercise and physical exertion can help reduce the threat of cancer and secondary cancers, particularly colon, bone, and cancer of the womb.

In addition, moderate and vigorous physical exertion is also supposed to be safe and helpful for numerous people with cancer.

There's strong substantiation that being active can help people with cancer, reduce passions of anxiety, ameliorate the quality of sleep, reduce fatigue, and boost energy situations.

Ameliorate fitness, strength, and physical exertion reduce depression, ameliorate lymphedema, which is a type of swelling caused by treatment of lymph bumps and generally ameliorate quality of life after cancer treatment.

There may be times during or incontinently after certain treatments that some types of exercise will need to be acclimated to or avoided for some people.

Some examples of this are for people who have low impunity following treatment, and they may need to avoid exercising in public places similar to gymnasiums with large numbers of people.

People who have had bone cancer will be advised to avoid placing too much stress on the bones and joints, so they may choose water-based conditioning as a safer option.

People who have had surgery similar to a mastectomy of the bone will need to take care of any arm movement or stress placed through the pectoral muscles, similar to doing press-ups, and people who have had lymph bumps removed will need to strike a balance with the volume and intensity of the exercise they do to avoid an overloaded lymphatic system, especially for the muscles near the point of the removed lymph bumps.

As a side note, if you've had surgery to remove lymph bumps from your crest, you should also wear your contraction sleeve while exercising if you've been given one to reduce the threat of lymphedema.

In all cases of witnessing care for cancer, it's important to get individual advice from your oncologist or croaker as to what they will recommend for you in the original stages over time, while in absolution, you can also bandy with an exercise specialist about the most applicable exercises for you're to get an acclimatized program to help you recover

. Trying to be physically active during certain types of cancer treatments can be incredibly grueling if you're currently having chemotherapy or radiotherapy.

The side goods during these types of treatments can make you feel veritably inadequately to the point that exercise may not indeed be on your radar it's veritably important that if you're having these particular treatments that the end of any physical exertion or exercise program is only to maintain your being fitness situations no progression should be tried during these stages of treatment because the curatives are so aggressive trying to ameliorate your fitness can be mischievous to your health as it'll complicate your symptoms of the adverse goods from the remedy thus remain as active as possible when you can which can be commodity as simple as getting out for a five nanosecond walk.

If you really do not feel well enough to do anything on a day during your treatment also do not as your body is telling you is trying to recover from it and this may vary day to day.

Some chemotherapy treatments are in cycles of three or four weeks and it may be that there are only a many days within each cycle that you feel well enough to do some form of physical exertion.

So, hear to your body and just doing a little bit when you can will make you feel more mentally and physically if you're witnessing hormonal or natural curatives also you may not feel relatively as inadequately as some other treatment types and you may find it easier to get into a habit of regular exercise but again only start when you feel ready and begin by being conservative and not setting yourself unrealistic pretensions.

Still, as with all cancer types, fatigue and frazzle are likely to be the overriding factors in your exercise capacity. Do not anticipate a gradual enhancement each week in your health and fitness, as there will be times when your exercise forbearance varies from day to day or week to week as you recover from the cancer and posterior treatments.

In terms of what you choose to do, make sure it's a commodity that you can manage, but more importantly, a commodity that you will enjoy, as this will help your adherence to it in the long term.

Swimming, or indeed gardening, can all be great ways of perfecting your situations of physical exertion without having to over-ply yourself.

CHAPTER SIX

POWER OF FACTORY-BASED DIET

The choices you make at the grocery store have a bigger impact than just your grand plans.

Filling your plate with foods that are grown on the ground may be a stylish diet for cancer prevention.

While some people have an advanced inheritable threat of developing cancer, exploration shows that nearly 25 percent of overall cancer cases could be averted with diet and nutrition alone.

Numerous cancers can take 10 or more years to develop, so everyday nutrition choices are pivotal in cancer prevention.

Factory-based diets are full of fruits, vegetables, and legumes, with little or no meat or other animal products. In exploration studies, insectivores, people who do not eat any animal products, including fish, dairy, or eggs, appeared to have the smallest rates of cancer of any diet.

The smallest rate was for insectivores, people who avoid meat but may eat fish or foods that come from creatures, such as milk or eggs.

Factory-ground foods do more than taste succulent. They're full of chemical composites, called phytochemicals, that protect the body from damage.

Phytochemicals also intrude on processes in the body that encourage cancer.

Factory-based diets are also high in fiber, which has been shown to lower the threat of bone and colorectal cancer.

Factory chemicals Phytochemicals offer numerous benefits.

In addition to guarding against damage, they drop inflammation and intrude on processes in the body that encourage cancer.

The most helpful phytochemicals are antioxidants.

This type of phytochemical protects the body from damage. Cancer grows when a cell's DNA is damaged. This causes abnormal cells to divide uncontrollably, which can insinuate and destroy normal body tissue.

Cell damage can also be caused by radiation, contagions, and exposure to other chemicals.

The body's natural metabolism creates oxidants that can cause cell damage as well. Antioxidants neutralize these damage processes while guarding and restoring cells.

Some foods that contain a high concentration of antioxidants include dark chocolate, apples with the peel, avocados, artichokes, red cabbage, tea, coffee, nuts, and grains. Carotenoids. These are fat-answerable composites, which means they need to be accompanied by a fat source to be absorbed.

Carotenoids are naturally present in numerous fruits, grains, canvases, and vegetables, such as carrots, sweet potatoes, squash, spinach, apricots, green peppers, and lush flora.

They're largely pigmented, so look for natural foods that are red, orange, unheroic, and green. Examples of carotenoids include beta-carotene, lycopene, and lutein. They've been linked to reducing the threat of heart disease, cancer, macular degeneration, and cataracts.

Numerous factory-ground foods are also high in provitamins called nascent and gamma-carotene. This nutrient is important for vision, growth, cell division, reduplication, and impunity.

Vitamin A also has antioxidant properties. Nutrients and phytochemicals set up in factory-ground foods feel the need to work together and singly to drop the cancer and complaint threat.

This means that factory-ground foods work best when eaten in combination with other foods rather than alone.

One prostate cancer study showed that a combination of tomato and broccoli diets was more effective at decelerating excrescence growth than either tomato or broccoli alone

FACTORY-GROUND FIBER

Factory-based diets are high in natural fiber. This has been shown to reduce cancer threats and moderate insulin situations.

Younger women who ate the most fiber-rich diets were 25 percent less likely to get bone cancer later in life. Other exploration finds that each 10 grams of diurnal fiber could lower the threat of colorectal cancer.

Healthy bacteria in the digestive tract can raise fiber and other beans to produce composites known to help promote normal colon development and reduce inflammation

. These bacteria convert some phytochemicals into further useable or active forms.

Eat for color and variety. There are numerous succulent options in a factory-based diet. trial with new fruits or vegetables or new ways to incorporate masses.

Cost can be a factor in opting for a factory-based diet menu, as fresh fruits and vegetables may be more precious.

Good druthers are frozen fruits and vegetables. They're flash-frozen to save nutrients and are less precious. Canned options are available, as well, for people with a stricter budget. Be sure to look for options without added sugar or swabs.

Aim to eat at least these quantities in your diet to feel full and get the necessary phytochemicals and fiber.

- Fruits: 1.5 to 2.5 mugs per day
- Vegetables: 2.5 to 4 mugs per day
- Whole grains, 3 to 5 ounces per day
- Legumes: 1.5 mugs per week
- Protein: 5 to 7 ounces per day
- Legumes, dairy, tofu, and eggs are excellent sources of protein. Or elect spare cuts of flesh and avoid reused flesh
- Fats: 3 to 5 servings per day. One serving equals one tablespoon of oil painting, four walnut halves, or one-sixth of an avocado.

Shifting to a factory-grounded diet

Eating a factory-grounded diet does not need to be all or nothing. Making gradual changes is more sustainable and realistic for most people.

Some ways to do this include: Start your day off right. Enjoy a succulent and healthy breakfast with whole-grain oatmeal, buckwheat, or quinoa, along with fruit, to give you the energy to attack your day.

Trial with meatless refections. "Meatless Mondays" and try one new meatless form per week. Treat meat like a seasoning. Instead of using meat as the main dish, use just a little for flavor

Use legumes for bulk. Drop the quantity of meat in some fashions by adding the quantity of sap, lentils, or vegetables. These foods fill more space on your plate, so you will not feel deprived.

Cover about half of your plate with fruits and vegetables for lunch and dinner.

CHAPTER SEVEN

STRESS MANAGEMENT AND ITS IPACT ON CANCER

It might feel normal to constantly worry and feel stressed out after entering a cancer opinion. After all, it's a stressful time in life. Still, exploration has shown that stress can negatively impact overall health issues.

Stress can affect internal health and impact the uptake of unhealthy actions. Studies have shown that people who witness habitual stress are frequently likely to show signs of depression, anxiety, gorging or undereating, and sedentary cultures.

Habitual stress can indeed beget physical affections such as headaches, wakefulness, and fatigue.

As if that isn't bad enough, recent findings also suggest that stress can contribute to the spread of cancer.

Habitual stress is different from everyday stress. It's normal and not inescapably dangerous to feel stressed out about a forthcoming deadline or while running late to work. Still, long-term stress(or habitual stress) can cause physical changes in the body.

While habitual stress has not yet been proven to increase the threat of developing cancer, it may affect the excrescence's capability to grow and spread. This is likely due in part to the release of norepinephrine.

Norepinephrine is a hormone associated with stress. In a series of trials, the excrescences of mice exposed to stressful situations (similar to insulation) were more likely to grow and spread.

Experimenters also found that bone cancer cases that reported using beta blockers had a better chance of surviving treatment without relapse than those who didn't report using beta blockers.

Luckily, relieving stress doesn't have to be a time-consuming, portmanteau-leveling trip to the gym.

Experimenters have studied a myriad of ways to offset the release of stress hormones, and most of them can be done from the comfort of home.

In a country where over 70 percent of adults report constantly feeling stressed out, there are numerous people who can profit from these simple stress-reducing techniques.

Do a high-intensity interval drill(HIIT)

Exercise is associated with the release of endorphins, or 'feel good' hormones. While all exercise is good for your body, the advanced-intensity exercises have been set up to release further endorphins.

Regular exercise can also help lower the body's stress hormones over time. Find a commodity to laugh about that is important, like exercise. Experimenters have found that horselaugh can also release endorphins.

Spending time with one's silliest musketeers or getting drawn into the depths of YouTube can be remedial when it comes to stress.

Talk it out occasionally

stress builds mountains out of operative hills. It can be especially delicate to de-stress when the brain is overwhelmed. Try talking it out with a loved one, or indeed in the glass.

Getting the negative studies out in the open can help the brain easily reuse them.

Take time for the effects you love.

Whether stress comes from feeling overbooked or dealing with changes, taking time to enjoy pursuits can ease the mind.

Making time for favorite conditioning is a simple way to show tone-love and help the body reduce stress.

Give and admit physical affection

Physical affection makes people feel loved, wanted, and safe. Along with soothing emotional benefits, there are also physiological changes that can reduce stress, along with physical affection.

Spend time outside

Getting fresh air and a cure for verdure can be incredibly relaxing and refreshing. Not unexpectedly, numerous studies have shown that the great outdoors is a great remedy for the passions of depression, anxiety, and stress.

The tranquility of nature balances out the continual stimulus that individuals experience in daily life and reduces stress as a consequence!

Play with a canine still, fresh air, and physical affection can reduce stress if exercised.

Limit alcohol, caffeine, and nicotine

Though frequently considered a stress-relieving vice, alcohol, nicotine, and caffeine frequently beget anxiety and wakefulness, which contribute to the body's stress response.

Clear your mind

One common reason people don't exercise the forenamed stress relievers is because they feel as if there isn't enough time.

Stress frequently tricks the brain into feeling overwhelmed and pressed for time. Luckily, clearing the mind and taking some deep breaths only require a couple of twinkles and can be done from anywhere.

Rehearsing contemplation at the start of the day, in the shower, at lunch, or before bed can greatly relieve stress. Seek professional help.

Still, it's important to speak with a croaker about these issues if habitual stress is snooping with everyday functions. A croaker may be suitable to recommend supplements, define drugs, or recommend a therapist to help with stress operations.

CHAPTER EIGHT

QUALITY SLEEP FOR A CANCER-RESISTANT BODY

Sleep plays a vital part in maintaining your health. When we think about how to take care of our overall health, we presumably consider healthy eating, regular exercise, and taking care of our internal health. But there are four, not three, areas that we need to consider

The thing we most take for granted is sleep. Prioritizing our sleep is a commodity, so numerous of us just don't do it, but it's well established that good sleep's essential for good overall health.

During sleep, your body repairs and regulates your cells, aprons, and muscles. At the same time, your brain processes studies, passions, and feelings that you've endured during the day.

Sleep boosts our vulnerable system, helps regulate our mood, and gives us the provocation to exercise, eat well, and go about our daily lives. So without good sleep, our bodies and minds can't and won't serve their purpose.

But when we talk about "good" sleep, what do we mean? Good sleep refers to quality sleep with a suitable duration. Getting 12 hours of poor sleep won't have the same salutary effects as eight hours of good-quality sleep.

How do you know if you're sleeping well? It's relatively simple if you wake up feeling well-rested and restored, with energy to get through the day, and your sleep quality is presumably good.

We know that poor sleep is linked to the development of diseases such as diabetes, cardiovascular disease, and rotundity. So it's not a huge step to assume that our sleep can also impact our risk of developing cancer. You don't have to live with poor sleep

. Numerous people don't realize that most sleep diseases respond really well to treatment. Sleepstation can help you identify the root cause of your poor sleep, produce a plan for you to follow, and support you in rebuilding your sleep. Fix your sleep.

Studies have looked at whether how long we sleep(long or short duration) or how well we sleep(sleep quality) can impact our risk of going on to develop cancer.

To probe the links between sleep and the cancer threat, experimenters frequently compare how long people sleep (i.e., sleep duration) with whether they also go on to develop cancer or not.

Most of these studies have looked at whether sleep duration, either short or long, could be associated with the threat of cancer. The results surely aren't clear-cut.

Numerous studies suggest that short sleep duration increases the threat of cancer, whereas some have discovered associations between certain cancers and long sleep duration. Other studies find no definite link at all between how long we sleep and our risk of cancer.

Recently, researchers examined data from nearly 24,000 people who signed up for a health exploration study. They looked at data collected from actors nearly eight times and compared their average sleep time at the launch of the study with whether they went on to develop cancer and other conditions.

Results showed that, compared to average sleep (7–8 hours per hour), short sleep (less than 6 hours per day) was associated with a greater than 40% increased threat of overall cancer.

In discrepancy, a meta-analysis (where the results of numerous studies are compared together) looked at the results from 65 studies and showed no overall increase in the threat of cancer overall.

There are studies that show associations between specific types of cancer and sleep duration, such as bone cancer and colorectal cancer.

But when we talk about "association," it means that people with the specific cancer had shorter sleep times than people who didn't have that cancer.

It doesn't mean that the short sleep time was the reason for developing the cancer. It could be a factor in the development of cancer, and, most probably, it's just one part of a more complex picture.

Inadequate sleep has been linked to the threat of cancer when looking at individual populations, terrain, or ethnic backgrounds. For illustration, in the meta-analysis bandied over, studies were grouped by the geographical locales of Europe, the USA, and Asia, and a link was set up between short sleep duration and cancer threat in the Asian population only.

In another study, the cohort was made up of uniquely Mexican-American actors, and the results showed an increased threat of cancer in actors who slept less than six hours per night.

The implicit reasons for certain populations having advanced threats aren't clear, but they could be due to differences in culture, life, genetics, or a blend of all three.

While it's not possible to generalize and say that sleep duration influences the cancer threat, we do know that inadequate sleep has a negative effect on overall health, so knowing you're sleeping well can only be a positive thing for your health.

Still, if you're floundering with a sleep problem, it's a good idea for your general health to try to address this if you feel like your sleep isn't optimal.

THE BIOLOGY OF SLEEP AND CANCER

When we talk of "cancer,, it's important to understand that it's not one distinct illness. According to Cancer Research UK, there are actually more than 200 different types of cancer.

Cancer is a marquee term for a huge number of different diseases that all affect the mortal body in their own way. The defining point that brings all cancers together is that they all beget the unbridled growth of cells within the body.

So given that the word cancer is used to define a large and different group of diseases, the relationship between sleep and cancer is also going to be complex.

Looking at the exploration data, it appears that certain cancers may be more caused by sleep than others. It's also reasonable to assume that, indeed, when two people have the same cancer type, one person's sleep may be disintegrated further than another.

Anyhow, regardless of the type of cancer studied, when looking at the natural links between sleep and cancer, exploration substantially focuses on three areas: dislocation of circadian measures, vulnerable function, and melatonin stashing. So we'll explore each of these three areas in a little further detail.

Numerous studies have established links between the body timepiece, circadian measures, and the development of cancer. But what exactly does all of this mean? Our body runs on a roughly 24-hour schedule, which we call our circadian meter.

This schedule is naturally synchronized to evening and daylight and is controlled by the body timepiece, which is the name given to specialized cells that make up a part of the brain called the suprachiasmatic nexus (SCN). The mortal body actually has numerous different timepieces that are responsible for timing regular events in the body.

All of these minor timepieces are under the control of the master timepiece in the brain. They control when certain chemicals in the body rise and fall, regulating a host of bodily functions to ensure that your body works as it should.

suppose the master timepiece is the head office, and all the lower timepieces are departments within the company(the body). The master timepiece responds to light and dark signals to keep all the lower timepieces in line. So, when we open the curtains in the morning and the sun sets in, light passes into our eyes, signals are sent to the SCN, and this leads to all of our timepieces being synchronized.

This is like head office transferring out memos to say,'It's day—let's get to work!'and each department also synchronizes its timepiece and starts its tasks. Jobs might include controlling our temperature, starting processes that we use during our waking hours, or stopping products that were demanded overnight but not during the day.

These measures are what keep the balance in our bodies and allow us to remain healthy and go about our daily lives with energy. Unfortunately, there are numerous effects that can disrupt that balance

. A simple illustration of this is jetlag. Flying across time zones can throw your body's circadian measures out of sync, and the result is that you can feel headachy, sick, or just not relatively right.

An analogous effect can occur when you don't get enough sleep or, indeed, when you sleep and wake up feeling sleepy.

These are short-term dislocations in your circadian meter, and they can be corrected by getting enough sleep at the right time of day.

Problems arise when these short-term disturbances become regular. If you're constantly at odds with your natural measures, the body is left trying to maintain balance amidst chaos.

Imagine head office transferring out its morning memo at 3 a.m. Or transferring out multiple copies of the morning memos throughout the day or at different times every day.

This is what we mean when we talk about the circadian meter being disintegrated. It's well known. The system will collapse as a result of confusion and disarray in every department.Tthat dislocation of our circadian measures is a threat factor for numerous different forms of cancer.

In our ultramodern, fast-paced world, we frequently keep to schedules that go against our natural circadian measures.

According to one study, 75 percent of the working population in industrialized countries works atypical hours(defined as outside of the 8 p.m. core hours).

So many of us stay up late, work irregular shift patterns, and rise at hours when we should typically be sleeping. By going against our natural circadian measures, we could intentionally be impacting our cancer threat.

Numerous studies have shown that long-term shift work can come with an advanced threat of cancers similar to those involving the bone, colon, ovaries, and prostate.

Still, when it comes to bone cancer and shift work, several large studies from 2021 have failed to find a link between shift work and cancer. So this association is surely not clear-cut.

Nevertheless, minimizing dislocation from our normal fleshly measures is a commodity we should all try to take on board, especially if you're a shift worker or work irregular hours.

We've got lots of tips to help shift workers sleep well, and general recommendations are that people who work shifts shouldn't overlook the significance of regular cancer wellness programs.

Keeping up with mammograms, having a prostate check, or making sure you carry out the recommended webbing for colorectal cancer can all help to identify cancers beforehand.

And this advice isn't limited to people who work shifts; earlier opinions can ameliorate success rates for the treatment of cancer.

Can circadian rhythms enhance the effectiveness of cancer treatment?

We've discussed how disturbances of our circadian rhythms caused by insufficient sleep, irregular sleeping habits, and work schedules may affect cancer, but there is also a more advantageous relationship between cancer and circadian rhythms.

According to studies, cancer patients with regular sleep and waking times had better results and a higher quality of life than those with erratic patterns and poor sleep.

This implies that by maintaining a daily pattern that includes going to bed at a decent hour, prioritizing sleep, and avoiding activities that interfere with our circadian rhythms, we are likely strengthening our defenses against cancer.

Melatonin

Investigating the connections between melatonin and cancer has drawn a lot of attention from the cancer research community. A hormone called melatonin is essential for making us feel drowsy.

Melatonin levels in the body are quite low all day. Melatonin production rises as the day progresses and darkness falls, which causes you to feel drowsy.

Melatonin, a hormone essential for making us feel drowsy, stops being produced when the morning sunshine streams into our eyes. We slow down melatonin synthesis in the morning, which prevents us from feeling tired.

We unknowingly expose ourselves to light sources that might disrupt our melatonin synthesis when we lengthen our days with artificial light, perhaps by spending our nights devoted to social media or absorbed in a TV series.

However, how does melatonin relate to cancer?

Melatonin has been discovered to possess a wide range of anticancer characteristics by scientific investigation. It has been shown to have anticancer benefits against malignancies of the skin, ovary, blood, and lungs.

On the other hand, those with lower melatonin levels actually have a greater chance of getting cancer.

Insufficient or interrupted sleep, exposure to artificial illumination, and other factors that might interfere with the circadian cycle can all lower melatonin levels..

This does not imply that we should all start taking melatonin right now. Melatonin should not be used without a doctor's supervision since it is a hormone that affects numerous bodily systems and is only accessible by prescription in many countries (including the UK and the European Union, Japan, Australia, and Canada).

Getting enough exposure to sunshine throughout the day is the best approach to maintaining appropriate melatonin levels. Reduce your exposure to bright lights and screens in the evening if you're resting or unable to go outdoors while receiving therapy.

Dark blinds or even black-out drapes may be beneficial in order to ensure that your bedroom is as dark as possible and encourage your brain to create melatonin.

Immune system

Our biological clock regulates when we sleep and wake up and is essential for enhancing immune performance.

Our immune system becomes more active when we are sleeping, and the body actually experiences greater amounts of inflammation than it does during the day.

The body clock controls when the concentrations of certain immune system chemicals increase and decrease.

Levels of immune molecules normally increase during the night to perform their responsibilities in these functions while we sleep, when our body is busy mending muscles and doing housekeeping duties to eliminate toxins and trash.

Sleep patterns that are delayed might mess with the body clock. When you routinely stay up late (for business or pleasure) and then sleep all day, your biological clock is thrown off, which causes chronic inflammation.

The biological clock sends signals throughout the night for inflammation levels to decline as repairs and maintenance are finished and your body prepares for a new day.

Your body clock will naturally desire to do these duties throughout the night while you are awake if you often stay up late or work the night shift.

Therefore, when you're working, socializing, or binge-watching Netflix, the body clock transmits signals that raise inflammation; these signals are most effective while the individual is sleeping.

Because sleep is the time for healing, when you go to bed at a time that doesn't correspond with your normal body rhythm, the body clock is more confused.

During the night, inflammatory chemicals that were previously elevated remain elevated in the body.

Overall, compared to people who sleep at times that are consistent with their natural body clock, inflammatory levels are consistently elevated in people who regularly have poor sleep or work nights.

One of the most often mentioned issues among cancer patients is sleep disruption.

Numerous studies have shown that sleep problems are a regular occurrence for cancer patients. For some patients, the sleep disruption may have started before their cancer diagnosis, but for others, it may have started after they learned they had cancer.

Many cancer patients have sleep issues during and after treatment. It is evident that sleep quality may be affected at any point throughout a cancer patient's journey. We'll examine each stage and potential factors impacting sleep.

Cancer symptoms may interfere with sleep.

For some individuals, sleep issues may start even before they've been given a cancer diagnosis, but they may also be a side effect of their malignancy.

Symptoms of a developing tumor might include a variety of things that make it difficult to sleep at night, such as digestive problems including nausea, vomiting, diarrhea, or constipation. Pain, breathing problems fever, itching, and bladder problems, extreme daily fatigue that necessitates naps and vague tumor-related pain.

Furthermore, even without being able to identify a particular cause, the growth of a tumor in the body might result in alterations that affect sleep patterns.

As a result, as you can see, the potential for developing sleep issues is often there even before a person is aware that they have cancer.

Being diagnosed with cancer is a life-altering and terrible event. It should come as no surprise that receiving this news will alter your mood and maybe interfere with your sleep. As a consequence of their diagnosis, many cancer patients may feel stress, anxiety, or despair.

We are aware of the significant connection between sleep and mental health and the benefits of getting enough sleep for our mental health. Therefore, optimizing your sleep may help to lessen symptoms of despair, anxiety, or stress if you're experiencing any of these..

At this point, you may want to establish a regular wind-down regimen for yourself. Maintaining a consistent schedule may aid in sleep and provide you with a sense of control during a period of great uncertainty.

After receiving a diagnosis, it's very natural to experience a wide range of emotional emotions, which may easily interfere with your nighttime sleep. While some may wake up throughout the night and have difficulty getting back asleep as they absorb their diagnosis, other individuals may have difficulty falling asleep.

It could be helpful to try using some thought-blocking tactics if you have trouble falling asleep, staying asleep, or waking up in the middle of the night.

It's critical that you don't just disregard your sleep. You will be able to unwind and sleep as a result or minimize them in light of a cancer diagnosis.

The best method to deal with sleep issues is to address them as soon as they appear, and establishing healthy sleep patterns as soon as possible following a diagnosis can only be advantageous.

Cancer therapies may interfere with sleep.

Each person's body will react differently to cancer since no two tumors are the same. The main reason there isn't a single "cure" for cancer is because of this. In actuality, every cancer is distinct and will react to therapy individually.

As a result, cancer therapies differ based on the patient as well as the kind of disease. All cancer therapies, however, have the potential to sporadically disrupt your sleep as a side effect.

One or more of the following methods will often be used in the treatment of cancer:

- Surgery
- Chemotherapy
- Immunotherapy
- radiation treatment

- hormone treatment.

It's typical to need some time to relax and recover after many of these therapies, which may include taking naps, going to bed earlier, or sleeping longer.

Even though these steps are vitally essential for the healing process, it's important to remember that once you feel better, you should strive to return to your usual sleeping schedule.

Continued irregular sleeping patterns, daytime naps, and nighttime snoozes may all support the formation of bad sleep patterns and lead to the onset of insomnia.

Let's go through each sort of therapy in greater depth and discuss how it could impact your ability to sleep.

Surgery

It's normal to have some fear and stress before any operation, and this may prevent you from sleeping in the days leading up to the procedure.

According to Brazilian research, being knowledgeable about the operation might help to lessen anxiety before cancer surgery.

Participants' anxiety levels were much lower when provided thorough information about their procedure in advance than when they were left in the dark.

This implies that it's probably beneficial to make sure you have all the facts to feel well-informed about the operation if you're getting ready for cancer surgery.

Knowing what to anticipate may make anxiety levels easier to control. Since anxiety and sleep are related, this may also help you sleep better in the days leading up to the event.

You can have trouble sleeping after cancer surgery while you're recovering. After surgery, your body will be working hard to heal and restore itself, which may interfere with sleep.

You can have pain or discomfort that keeps you up at night or worry about how the procedure went.

It has been shown that sleep may affect how surgeries turn out.

People who have trouble sleeping the night before surgery run the risk of having a longer recovery period and more severe post-operative discomfort, nausea, and vomiting.

In contrast, getting the best possible sleep at this time is crucial for a speedy recovery. After surgery, getting a good night's sleep helps hasten healing, lessen swelling, and hasten recovery.

Examining your bedroom's layout before surgery will help make sure it's ready for a peaceful recuperation when you come home.

It is important to take into account how your hospital stay may affect your sleep if you will be recuperating in a hospital.

In general, hospitals are bustling, bright, and loud. You could find that using earplugs or an eye mask to filter out the light can help you sleep better while in the hospital.

Even packing your favorite pillow, blanket, or book for bedtime might be a good idea for your trip.

Radiation treatment, chemotherapy, and immunotherapy

The goal of therapy with these medicines is to eradicate the invasive cancer cells. Your body must work very hard to get rid of all the ensuing dead cells, which may have a significant impact on your ability to fall asleep.

Additionally, these therapies' adverse effects might cause issues including headaches, nausea, discomfort, or an upset stomach. Your sleep may be disturbed by any of these.

Fortunately, there are several drugs you may use to reduce discomfort during and after these therapies.

You can regulate how well you sleep throughout this period, even if you can't forecast or control how your body will react to these treatments. You may attempt a variety of easy sleep practices on your own to see if you can improve your sleep while undergoing therapy.

Even apparently insignificant strategies, like practicing excellent sleep hygiene, creating a relaxing bedtime ritual, and reducing screen time in the evenings, might help you sleep better while undergoing treatment.

Hormone therapies

Medication that specifically targets key hormone pathways is also used to treat a number of malignancies. Our body's natural hormonal pathways may be changed, and this can have a significant impact on how well we sleep.

People often describe night sweats as one of the symptoms that disturb their sleep after hormone therapy, which is frequently used to treat breast and prostate cancer.

It may be beneficial to keep your bedroom a little cooler at night if your therapy includes hormone medications, and choosing cotton or linen sheets and nightclothes may help drain moisture from the body.

In addition to your main prescription throughout treatment, you could also be given painkillers, steroids, antibiotics, or nausea-relieving drugs. Many of these medications may disrupt sleep.

Regardless of the treatment plan, your medical team will be aware that certain medications or drug combinations might disrupt sleep. As a result, these medications are often administered at specified times of the day to minimize their potential impact on sleep.

If your therapy is affecting your ability to sleep, it's crucial that you let your doctor know. There are many choices available to assist you in improving your sleep, so don't suffer in silence. Effective sleep is essential for effective recovery.

Post-treatment

After therapy is done, the body's recuperation process lasts for some time. There is no set period of time for recovery from cancer, and each person will experience physical and mental recovery at a different pace.

Many cancer survivors have emotional difficulties as a result of anxieties about recurrence, progression, or survivor guilt even after completing treatment, entering remission, and receiving the all-clear.

Cancer survivors are said to have greater levels of despair, stress, and anxiety, and we know that our mental health and sleep quality may interact in significant ways.

It's a sad truth that many individuals who have had cancer treatment report having trouble sleeping, and we are aware that cancer survivors have high rates of insomnia.

As we've already discussed, sleeplessness may be a sign of cancer both before and after a diagnosis, as well as during and after therapy. It is not unexpected that many cancer patients who have completed their treatment have sleeplessness.

Cancer-related insomnia may last for years after treatment is finished, and cancer survivors have significantly more difficulty sleeping than the general population does.

Even though there is ample evidence that patients who have cancer have considerably greater rates of insomnia and sleep disruption, sleep is still often ignored in cancer treatment settings.

Cancer survivors may attempt to live with their sleep issues or search for methods to self-manage their symptoms since there aren't enough programs accessible to help them.

CHAPTER NINE

DETOXFICATION AND CLEANSING

Chemical poisons generated by the body during regular metabolism as well as environmental contaminants are continually present in our bodies.

If the body is unable to adequately cleanse itself, the buildup of toxins often results in cellular damage and inflammation, which increases the chance of developing major chronic illnesses like cancer..

Pesticides, metals, toxic chemicals, environmental pollutants, synthetic food additives, poisons, and chemical waste created internally are just a few examples of the many things that are poisonous to the body.

Why do toxins build up in the body?

The body may get polluted with toxins by being exposed to environmental contaminants such as heavy metals, pollution, tainted water and food, excessive alcohol consumption, pollution, smoking, cigarette usage, pharmaceutical medications, toxic chemicals, and infectious illnesses.

Additionally, internal stress, nasty bacteria, yeast, and viruses may emit toxic substances.

DETOXIFICATION

The process of detoxification involves removing and purging poisons from the body. A detoxification program's goal is to stop and undo cellular damage, which poses major health concerns otherwise.

Many symptoms and diseases are improved by getting rid of extra pollutants. Typically, natural side effects include improved skin and weight reduction.

Effective detoxification improves overall welfare, health, energy, and vigor. For cell regeneration and lifespan, frequent detoxification regimens are essential.

What natural detoxification processes does the body have?

The capacity for self-detoxification is built into the human body. The body really has a number of processes in place for getting rid of waste.

The skin, liver, lungs, large intestine, and kidneys are the primary organs that make up the waste elimination system. However, for a variety of reasons, natural detoxification may not completely remove toxins from the body.

Major detoxification pathways, including those in the blood, gut, and lymph, are crucial to maintaining a healthy balance between sickness and wellbeing.

What results in a buildup of toxins in the body?

Exposure to pollutants over an extended period of time, stress, and bad lifestyle choices.

Do we create some of the poisons we consume?

Yes. Some poisons are produced inside as a result of stress, unfavorable thoughts, and unrestrained emotions.

Additionally, bacterial imbalance or invasion by foreign species may produce harmful waste.

What methods of detoxification are there?

In the paradigm of integrative health care, there are several detoxification regimens available. You may use the following techniques to get rid of toxins in your body:

- Exercise/movement (yoga, meditation, breathing exercises, and prayer)
- Alkaline or pure water
- Diet
- Fasting
- Juicing Additives
- Massages and body scrubs for detox
- Radiant-heat sauna
- The lymphatic system
- Autohemotherapy (ozone treatment)
- IV detoxification
- Aquatic Colon Therapy
- Osteopathy

Does detoxification lower the risk of cancer?

To reduce pollutants and advance health, it is crucial to give our bodies the rest they need, move about, sweat, drink enough pure water, consume foods rich in fiber and water content (such as fruits and vegetables), and engage in other healthy lifestyle habits.

Our body automatically detoxifies itself by removing accumulated waste products each day.

The illness process starts when cells begin to malfunction as a result of free radicals, a byproduct of inflammation, and the body's capacity to eliminate toxic waste is insufficient compared to the toxic overload.

To get rid of too many toxins and the dangers they pose to your body, detoxification is essential.Based on the idea that an excess of toxins significantly contributes to cellular damage and disease development, cancer risk may be prevented and perhaps reversed by removing toxins from the body.

CONCLUSION

The "The Anti-Cancer Lifestyle" book's core themes include making morally right decisions and hoping for a better, cancer-resistant future.

It represents a lifetime dedication to one's health and well-being. One gains the knowledge and abilities needed to take control of their health and cancer prevention

. Being a captain requires one to seek out new knowledge, be open to investigation, and modify one's lifestyle choices. The knowledge inspires people to lead cancer-free lifestyles by being shared with family and friends.

This journey isn't just for one person; instead, it's a part of a larger effort to create a society where cancer is less common and everyone has access to exceptional health.

www.ingramcontent.com/pod-product-compliance
Lightning Source LLC
Chambersburg PA
CBHW060956260726
48661CB00005B/1898